A

CHINESE AND WESTERN DAILY
PRACTICAL HEALTH GUIDE

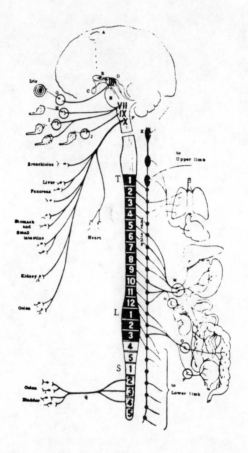

Plan of the Autonomic Nervous System. Parasympathetic fibers on left, sympathetic fibers on right. (From Best and Taylor).

A CHINESE
AND
WESTERN
DAILY PRACTICAL
HEALTH GUIDE

BY

BETTY YÜ-LIN HO
RESEARCH DIRECTOR

NEW YORK
JUVENESCENT RESEARCH CORPORATION
1982

Library of Congress Cataloging in Publication Data

Ho, Betty Yü-Llin
     A Chinese and Western daily practical health guide.

     Includes bibliographical references.
     1. Health.   2. Body, Human.   3. Medicine, Popular.
1. Title.
     RA776.5. H578   613   81-20848
     ISBN 0-9600148-4-5   AACR2

TO

AMANDA, ANITA, RAOUL

AND

TO THE MEMORY OF

JULIEN

Quant au mystère . . . . ,
un homme ici a tracé la seule
voie, par où un **philo**sophe
sérieux puisse passer-un homme, le plus grand parmi nous:
Blaise Pascal.*

Constant Bourquin

*As for the mystery.......... one man here has marked out the
only course a serious philosopher must take - one man, the
greatest among us: **Blaise** Pascal.
(Translated by B. Y-L Ho.)

ABOUT THE AUTHOR

Betty Yü-Lin Ho is born in China.
Educated at the Lycée Français in Shanghai, she later obtained a B.S. in Biology from Columbia University in New York City. In 1955 she attended a year of medical school at Lausanne University in Switzerland. Abandoning medicine for serious studies at the piano, it was during her musical studies that many scientific hypotheses came to her.

From 1958 to 1965 Betty Yü-Lin Ho developed an infant feeding method which has since, obtained both Canadian and U.S. patents. Research begun in 1963 to prove her hypotheses led to the writing of eight scientific books. In the present 9th guide, the author presents her ideas to the public in a nutshell.

Research director of a non-profit medical research organization, the author, who resides in New York City, is at present in the process of writing her 10th manuscript.

TABLE OF CONTENTS

Part II. PRACTICAL SUGGESTIONS ATTAINED BY EXPERIMENTAL REASONING UPON ESTABLISHED SCIENTIFIC FACTS.

TABLE OF CONTENTS

ILLUSTRATIONS

PREFACE

In 1939 famed surgeon Alexis Carrel felt the need for a scientific guide to help direct man's life in our present mechanized, industrialized society.

The English neurologist Sir Russel Brain delivered a speech in 1953. He stressed the importance of a philosophy of life, the intuitive ability to see in the whole something more than just the sum of its parts. He felt that such intuitive ability required a broader education in the humanities rather than routine training in a medical school. To him this combination is a prerequisite to arrive at a philosophy of medicine.

Author Betty Yǔ-Lin Ho, research director of a nonprofit medical research organization, has written 8 scientific books. Fluent in seven languages, violinist and accomplished pianist, the author presents her scientific ideas here, in a nutshell, The directions given were arrived at through experimental reasoning upon established scientific facts collected over a period of 19 years.

ACKNOWLEDGEMENTS

The author wishes to thank the following for permission to use illustrations in her book.

Plan of the Autonomic Nervous System, from THE LIVING BODY, 4th Edition, by Charles H. Best and Norman B. Taylor. Copyright 1938, © 1944, 1952, © 1958 by Holt, Rinehart and Winston, Inc. Copyright © 1966 by Charles H. Best and Norman B. Taylor. Reprinted by permission of Holt, Rinehart and Winston, Inc.

Evolution of the facial angle, from THE HUMAN SKELETON, AN INTERPRETATION, by H.E. Walter, 1918. Reprinted by permission of Mrs. Alice Walter Fulton.

Preparations from vitally injected muscles from guinea pig. Optical transverse sections. The muscle capillaries of guinea pig injected during life with India ink showing different degrees of constriction. From ANATOMY AND PHYSIOLOGY OF CAPILLARIES, revised edition, 1929, by August Krogh. Reprinted by permission of Yale University Press.

Series of 5 drawings illustrating the stages of growth from the end of the 3rd week to the end of the 8th, from A. Keith's HUMAN EMBRYOLOGY AND MORPHOLOGY. Reprinted by permission of Mr. H.M. Evans.

Figure 8 (P. 78) and Figure 10 (p. 89). From NEW PATHS IN BIOLOGY by Adolf Portmann. Translated by Arnold J. Pomerans. Planned and edited by Ruth Nanda Anshen. World Perspectives Series, Vol. 30. Copyright © 1964 by Harper & Row, Publishers, Inc. Reprinted by permission of the publishers.

INTRODUCTION

In order to be able to control your body at all times, to understand why under given conditions it will react a certain way, to master your functions at will even under dire conditions of health, it is necessary to have a completely different outlook about your body.

The sole reason why it has been so difficult to solve the various vital problems mankind is faced with continuously is due to the fact that modern medicine has not been able to view the living body functioning as whole.

The present daily guide intends to present the body working as a whole with practical suggestions to help you direct yourself during a lifetime.

PART I

HOW
THE BODY
FUNCTIONS AS A WHOLE

CHAPTER I

HOW YOU MUST VIEW THE LIVING BODY

You must consider your body as being made up of 6 functioning systems, where the regulatory organs represent the motor and the remaining 5 systems are the active working parts.

These 6 organ - systems are, namely:

1. The regulatory organs and their glands.
2. The reproductive organs and their glands.
3. The digestive organs and their glands.
4. The sex organs and their glands.
5. The muscles and bones and their glands.
6. The sense organs and their glands.

CHAPTER II

HOW THE SIX SYSTEMS ARE UNITED

The 6 organ - systems are united by the blood whose flow is controlled by the three great nerve centers:
The brain.
The sympathetic ganglia.
The parasympathetic ganglia.

These 3 nerve centers are tied together in their function by the spinal cord.

CHAPTER III

HOW THE THREE NERVE CENTERS CONTROL
THE SYSTEMS

Of the three nerve centers, each controls two systems.

The Brain Controls:

The muscles and bones and their glands and the sense organs and their glands *

The Sympathetic ganglia control:

The regulatory organs and their glands and the reproductive organs and their glands.

The Parasympathetic ganglia control:

The sex organs and their glands and the digestive organs and their glands.

* The sense organs are also automatically controlled.

CHAPTER IV

WHERE NERVE CENTERS EFFECT THEIR CONTROL

The nerve centers control the systems at the level of their capillaries. The 3 great nerve centers send tiny end fibers to the minute capillary beds of the 6 systems.

Whenever a vital function is performed oxygen is delivered at capillaries. This continuous supply of oxygen enables us to perform our manifold life processes.

The tiny nerve end-fibers allow a capillary area to open up, whereby blood flows to the area in greater quantity. This increased supply of blood delivers more oxygen to maintain the greater metabolism which activity necessitates.

The tiny nerve end-fibers also restrict a capillary area thereby lessening blood flow to the organ. This happens whenever an active organ is relaxed or inactive.

CHAPTER V

HOW THE NUMBER OF CAPILLARIES CAN BE AFFECTED

Work and rest affect the number of open capillaries in an organ.

In an active organ, many capillaries are open, thus letting red blood cells flow through them in large quantities.

On the contrary many capillaries are closed when an organ is inactive, in this fashion restricting the passage to red blood cells.

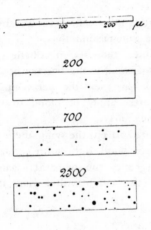

Fig. 1. Preparation from vitally injected muscles fron guinea pig.
Optical transverse sections(From Krogh)
You will notice that many more capillaries are open during heavy activity. In inactivity many capillaries are closed.

CHAPTER VI

HOW NERVE CENTERS EFFECT THEIR CONTROL ON CAPILLARIES

The tiny end fibers supplied by the three great nerve centers either voluntarily or involuntarily supply more or less blood to a capillary region. Thus:

The brain supplies more blood to a capillary area whenever active movement or sense perception is required.

As example, when you pick up an object, you open your hand. Your brain immediately enables a greater flow of blood to the opened capillaries of your hand, whereby more oxygen is delivered and you are able to hold the object.

The two other nerve centers control the various organ systems in the same fashion, thus:

During a meal the parasympathetic ganglia allow a larger supply of blood to the digestive organs.

When you have sex the parasympathetic ganglia enable a greater supply of blood to the sex organ, resulting in the climax.

When you fall asleep, the sympathetic ganglia direct a greater flow of blood to the entire regulatory organs.

During pregnancy, the sympathetic ganglia automatically supply the womb with a good flow of blood.

CHAPTER VII

WHAT HAPPENS TO BLOOD FLOW WITHIN THE SIX SYSTEMS

While blood automatically flows to a region whenever it becomes active, blood within a set of communicating tubes, flows according to Pascal's principle where if the liquid rises in 1 tube, it will be depleted from the other tubes. The sum of the depletions always equals the rise within the 1 tube.

If you were to parallel the 6 organ - systems of the living body with the 6 communicating tubes, you can see that no matter how the 6 organ-systems are juggled about, the regulatory organs suffer the greatest depletion of blood during a 24 hour day, for it is during sleep alone, lasting around 8 hours, that the regulatory organs receive the greatest supply of blood.

During the remaining hours of the day, they truly are being taxed.

While a decent blood supply is needed within the motor for smooth functioning of bodily parts, a better understanding can help us control this supply, for life. For example we can control the number of active systems at work so that the regulatory organs will not become depleted unnecessarily.

In general blood will flow to a region whenever it becomes active. As soon as it becomes inactive, at rest or relaxed, more blood will become available to supply another active region.

Total relaxation of the 5 active organ-systems will allow a great supply of blood to fill up the entire regulatory organs.

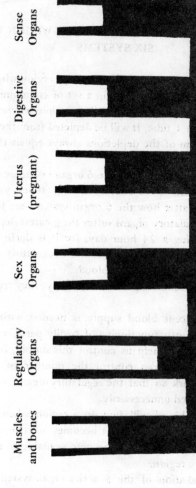

Fig. 2. Schematic representation of the six systems as six connected tubes where 5 systems are at work. Note how the regulatory organs are depleted.

A few systems at work

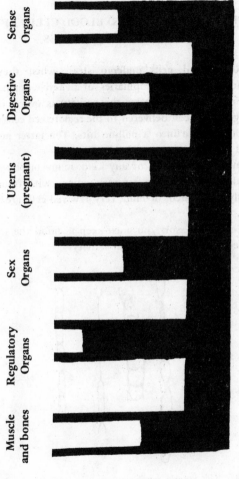

Fig. 3.   Schematic representation of the six systems when only a few systems are engaged in mild activity. The regulatory organs are slightly depleted.

CHAPTER VIII

WHAT HAPPENS TO RED BLOOD CELLS AFTER LEAVING CAPILLARIES

Red blood cells undergo stress when they pass through the opened capillaries of an active organ.

For this reason, after the activity is over with and oxygen has been delivered to the region, red cells literally disintegrate into a million bits. The latter are later used up to form more red cells.

In forceful action of any kind, many more red cells are destroyed. On the contrary, when a vital function is gently performed, or mild, very few red cells are destroyed.

For this reason you must keep in mind the strength of performance of your vital activity.

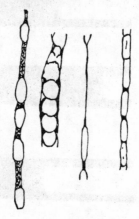

Fig .4. The muscle capillaries of guinea pig injected during life with India ink, showing diferent degrees of constriction (from Krogh)

CHAPTER IX

HOW CAPILLARIES THEMSELVES CAN BE AFFECTED

As red cells force their way through opened capillaries, rapidly delivering oxygen to maintain the increased metabolism of the active region, the walls of these tiny blood vessels can become greatly extended.

When this happens, vessel walls will bulge or even burst. This will diminish the number of tiny blood vessels of a region. In turn the metabolism of an area will be lessened.

It is especially true that when vessel walls are brittle as in arteriosclerosis, vessel walls can burst.

Particularly dangerous are any type of forced activity, driving red blood cells in clumps through opened capillaries.

Only unforceful action during a lifetime will preserve body capillaries indefinitely.

CHAPTER X

ACTIVITY AND TOTAL BLOOD VOLUME

Because so many red blood cells are destroyed after their passage through capillaries, vital activity can affect total blood volume when large capillary regions are involved.

For this reason it is good to analyze your daily activities and make sure no needless expenditure of energy is made during the waking hours.

You must be particularly wary of forced activity involving large capillary regions, i.e. muscles and bones, or where much energy is expended, as in operatic singing. You must be in perfect health to be able to perform such strenuous activity without detrimental effects.

When total blood volume is considerably lessened, your sleep may become light, impaired or simply disturbed. As time passes, the regulatory functions of the motor will become impaired.

You must remember that an average human being has around 5 liters of blood in his circulatory system.

CHAPTER XI

HOW TO EVALUATE VITAL MANIFESTATIONS

Vital manifestations will adversely affect the motor because total blood volume lessens after activity is over For this reason it is good to be able to assess the size of capillary regions, whether a single organ is used or an entire system is involved.

Muscles and bones represent 50% of total body weight. Excess activity involving muscles and bones and their vital manifestations can have a definite detrimental effect upon total blood volume.

When in full activity, the digestive system alone can contain the total blood volume.

The sex organs and reproductive organs lie dormant when inactive but in full activity, i.e. during the climax and during pregnancy, a large quantity of blood is utilized.

The sense organs are small in size, but the eyes and ears are continuously being stimulated by sights and sounds. Continuous exposure to stimuli can destroy a considerable amount of red cells.

From the above we can say that a system is large when a set of organs is in full activity. But when mildly active, dormant or when size of active organ is small, a system is said to be small.

CHAPTER XII

VITAL MANIFESTATIONS OF THE 6 ORGAN-SYSTEMS

Our various life processes are externally shown by manifestations of the 6 organ - systems.

Thus:

Manifestations of muscles and bones:

Talking, singing, murmuring, laughing, crying, walking, jogging, jumping, limping, running, climbing, carrying, etc.

Manifestations of the sense organs:

Seeing, hearing, tasting, smelling, touching, pressing, burning, freezing, pricking, itching, hurting, etc.

Manifestations of the reproductive organs:

Menstruation, conception, abortion, pregnancy, etc.

Manifestations of the digestive organs: Chewing, biting, swallowing, digestion, breath, salivation, hunger, pains, elimination, constipation etc.

Manifestations of the sex organs:

Libidinous sensations, erection, impotence, climax, ejection, etc.

Manifestations of the regulatory organs:

Breathing, pulse beat, perspiration, color and condition of skin, urine, sleep, etc.

The passions affecting the soul:

Pain, joy, ecstasy, fear, fright, meanness, anger, greed, sorrow, envy, fatigue etc.

CHAPTER XIII

SIZE OF ORGANS AND
VITAL MANIFESTATIONS

The potential capillary capacity of an organ is shown by its size. Thus the brain is roughly the size of a basketball or football, representing around two quarts of liquid.

Two legs represent at least 3 quarts of blood. Both hands, when active, represent at least 1/2 a quart of fluid.

The size of an organ shows how much blood is being used when it is active, and how the motor is being depleted.

In general mental activity is extremely strenuous as 2 quarts of blood are constantly in use. If you are weak constant mental activity can cause pyorrhea with loss of teeth, constipation, to end even in cancer. It is better not to do too much mental work during a lifetime.

If you are obliged to use your brain, make sure lights are dim, no sound disturbs you, that you recline your body as much as possible and make sure you sip something while you work.

PART II

PRACTICAL SUGGESTIONS ATTAINED BY
EXPERIMENTAL REASONING UPON
ESTABLISHED SCIENTIFIC FACTS

CHAPTER XIV

HOW TO AVOID GREAT DEPLETIONS OF
BLOOD FROM YOUR REGULATORY ORGANS

Alway sit up slowly upon awakening, rising slowly out of your bed.

Do not sleep under disturbed conditions of continuous noise, bright lights, chatter, loud music.

Do not wake a person up in a sudden: clanging bell, pail of cold water, telephone ring, shaking, etc.

Avoid speaking for a good half hour upon awakening. Begin the day by doing things at a slow pace.

Avoid loud, continuous talk, loud singing.

Do not holler across an adjoining room.

Do not speak above the din of machinery.

Use a bell to convey people for meals or other event.

Avoid noisy, crowded, bright environments after a day's work.

Try to use few organ-systems during the day.

Never use 2 or 3 organ-systems forcefully at once, i.e. shout upon a full stomach while standing on your feet; have sex after a day of physical exertion where you have had heavy meals, etc.

At best try to use 1 organ-system while keeping others in mild activity, i.e. use a dim light, keeping music down to bare audibility when doing concentrated mental work, seated on a high-back chair where you can recline your head, etc.

Make sure you have at least one bowel movement a day, if not more.

Avoid sex when heading for a long drive.

Plug your ears during the passage of a speedy express train.

Never frighten anyone or allow someone to frighten you.

Choose living quarters far from a rumbling highway, the train station, landing planes.

Travel to only one distant place in any day.

Do not look at rapidly moving cars.

Do not look at tall buildings.

Be sure to spit out a mouthful of boiling liquid, regardless of the occasion.

CHAPTER XV

HOW TO MAINTAIN OPTIMUM FUNCTION OF YOUR SKELETAL MUSCULATURE

Avoid expenditure of excessive physical energy.

Weight-lifting one of the best types of muscular exerttion.

Household chores recommended.

Long walks are excellent.

Natural fibers for clothing most conducive to health.

Knitted clothing, molding the body, are just about the best.

A flowing top hiding waistline enables greater relaxation.

Don a hat for yet greater relaxation.

Low-heeled mocassins provide satisfaction and allow control of food intake.

Avoid constricting brassieres and corsets.

Never exert 2 organ-systems forcefully: rapid sex and rapid meals, constant standing and much talking, etc.

Silence is of gold.

CHAPTER XVI

HOW TO MAINTAIN OPTIMUM FUNCTION OF YOUR DIGESTIVE SYSTEM.

Indulge in company for meals only once in a while.

Solitary meals most peace inducing.

Complete silence and dim lights should be the custom at mealtime.

Recline your body and head.

Let hands and arms hang relaxed on armchair especially during chewing and swallowing.

Pick at foods as much as possible.

Avoid large chunks of meat if possible.

Small pieces of food stimulate rapid digestion.

Make sure the bolus of food is as soft as mush before swallowing.

Alternate solid foods with a drink, always.

Use a straw to drink as much as possible.

Liquid foods are easiest to digest.

Solids come next. Fats are the hardest to dispose of.

Deep fried foods are to be eaten sparingly.

Dried starches soaked in a liquid are to be avoided at all costs.

Wet starches like pasta are healthier than dry starches, bread, cake.

Steamed starches are better than baked starches.

Wheat starch made into a dough to wrap up meats, etc. is most digestible.

Never eat a meal when in pain or in anger.

After a lengthy trip or when tired, always rest before your meal.

If possible, either listen to or play your favorite music after mealtime.

Soup taken after a meal or at mealtime helps daily regularity.

As much as possible let your hunger pains direct your desire to eat.

Never eat much beyond the point of fullness.

CHAPTER XVII

HOW TO MAINTAIN OPTIMUM FUNCTION OF
YOUR SEX ORGANS

Always allow your feelings to direct you in the choice of a mate.

Never allow yourself to be lured by a one-sided romance.

Sometimes acceptance is necessary.

Keep eyes and ears open for a lifetime partner between ages 15 and 25.

After 25 years of age extreme care must be exercised in the choice of a partner.

Falling in love ensures an optimum bed mate, but it must be on both sides.

For great sexual pleasure, have sex upon an empty digestive tract.

Have sex in the dark and in silence.

Avoid rapid accomplishment of the sex act.

Allow sex organs to lubricate fully by much foreplay to induce great sexual pleasure.

Only great lubrication ensures potency of sex organs for life.

Always try a patner our before engaging yourself in vows.

Self-improvement can turn a one-sided romance into a mutual relationship.

Self-improvement may involve body cleanliness, internal or external. A light diet, partial fasting, can help.

Better avoid the climax when sex organ is dry.
Better have a mate than practice masturbation.
Better go whithout sex than masturbate.
Practice sex sparingly in winter months.
Creative activity of any kind waives the need for sex.
Wear flowing, soft pants, skirts to avoid rubbing with hard clothing, to prevent sexual desires.
Remember that 1/2 a glass of blood is lost after a climax.
Playing a musical instrument can waive the need for sex.
Tighten up the entire abdominal region just before the climax.
Stimulate several mucous surfaces to provide great pleasure during climax.

CHAPTER XVIII

HOW TO MAINTAIN OPTIMUM FUNCTION OF YOUR REPRODUCTIVE ORGANS

Liquids should comprise greater proportion of your diet.

Practice sex sparingly.

Avoid constant loud talking.

As much as possible pick at your foods, much like a pigeon.

Practice occasional fasting when approaching menopause.

Sound sleep is very important.

Cut up your foods in bits before cooking.

Ever so often relax your body completely during the day.

Avoid all conditions that can cause tension.

Never allow your hands and feet to remain cold any length of time.

CHAPTER XIX

HOW TO CONCEIVE NORMALLY

Avoid sex particularly during the first 2 months of pregnancy.

Relax skeletal musculature as much as possible.

Do not knit or sew.

Avoid rapid gulping of foods.

Have as much fresh air as possible.

Avoid plane rides or other speedy trips.

Avoid tension at card games or other gambling.

Avoid looking down from a great height.

Avoid loud pounding noises as in construction or a speedy highway.

A peaceful atmosphere without commitments and worry is most conducive to a successful pregnancy.

Avoid drugs, smoking, alcohol.

Stay away from any environment that can cause infectious disease with high fever.

Sometimes it may be necessary to remain reclined during 9 months.

Avoid overexertion in all other four active organ-systems.

CHAPTER XX

HOW TO MAINTAIN OPTIMUM FUNCTION OF
YOUR REGULATORY ORGANS

Work in an environment of fresh air.

Have at least 2 hours of fresh air and sunshine daily.

Eat only when assailed with hunger pains.

Do not overfill youself at each meal.

Practice a day of fasting or skip the evening meal
when hunger pains are not powerful.

Do not run or jog excessively after age 20.

Never run uphill or up a flight of steps. Always climb up
slowly.

Avoid direct sunshine on bare skin.

Perspire when fully dressed in the summer to waive
illness in winter.

Ever so often, take your pulse at awakening. 2 beats per
inhalation is normal. 3 beats per inhalation denotes
fever.

Make sure your urine is always yellow, of s distinctive
smell.

Practice occasional fasting when your urine is white for
long perods.

Make sure your skin is smooth and silky.

Never eat food by the pound or in large quantities.

Allow your body to be shaken up in a subway, bus, or
carriage and sleep.

Silence and solitude maintain regulatory organs in optimum function.

Be moderate in all bodily activities.

Perspiration during sleep ensures continued proper function of motor.
Always sip a little dilute tea during the day. When travelling, bring some grapes with you or a drink.

CHAPTER XXI

HOW TO PRESERVE YOUR SENSE ORGANS

Use several 25 Watt pink bulbs with a fabric over parchment shade in all rooms.

Make sure TV screen is on dark side.

Never work under a bare bulb.

Use a yellow bulb, 5 or 10 Watts, in refrigerator.

Make sure TV sound is slightly above audibility when in use.

Learn to use rubber ear plugs whenever loud or continuous noise disturbs you, i.e. at typewriter, in subways, buses, planes, when driving, even during sleep if necessary.

Remove wax from ears, daily.

Look far into the distance as much as possible.

Stay in a silent environment whenever possible.

Avoid direct sunshine on bare skin.

Greasy foods are to be sparingly eaten.

Liquids are more important than solid foods, anytime.

Wear dark glasses when in an environment of neon lights. Especially important is the use of dim lighting for close work.

When light is too dim, you will experience discomfort in eyes.

You can quickly sense how much lighting you need for close work, without feeling discomfort or strain.

Never turn a radio on to a blasting level .

Tighten your eyes to a tight tremolo when you suddenly go from darkness into a bright place.

CHAPTER XXII

GENERAL BODILY CARE FOR GOOD HEALTH

Bathing and washing in general: Always gradually increase the hot water level. Never penetrate a tubful of hot water. Soap and scrub until no dirt rubs off and a loud noise is made upon passing fingers over skin.(About 1/2 hour).

Ears: Fifteen minutes after bathing, use an earpicker* to remove wax from ears. Learn to use an ear picker by scraping outside of ear first. Gradually penetrate deeper and deeper. Earpicking must be done in complete silence in a reclined position.

Clean ears removes the tendency to talk incessantly. You will then remain quiet 24 hours daily. It will help you save your energy and thus prolong your life.

Navel: Clean navel out daily.

Hair: Hair must always be washed with soap first, then with a shampoo. Never tie your hair in braids unless for short moments. Even an over all 2 inch long hairdo is damaging to health.

Men must adopt long hair, at least neck length, while women should never braid hair in tiny braids.

---

* Earpickers come in wood, bone, metal. They may be purchased for around a dollar in any gift shop in Chinatown.
Silver earpickers scrape deeply with a good scratching effect.
They cost around $3.00. Get a few different ones, one may work better than another.

Once in a while, take hold of a handful of hair and give it a tight pull. Do it for all your hair.

Teeth: Use a hard brush. Placing brush at junction of teeth and gums, massage in a circular motion.

Use a rubber tip for a quick massage between teeth, on both sides, in and out.　　Once in a while, tighten your teeth to a tight GRRR...

CHAPTER XXIII

HOW TO EXERCISE DURING A LIFETIME

On-the-spot exercise is best, i.e. jump, jog on the spot, pedal a bike, bend, stretch, pull, etc.

Strenuous exercise requiring the covering of distance is good only for those under age 25.

Long distance walks are excellent to induce perspiration in summer.

Weight lifting is one of the best forms of exercising.

Stretch, pull, tighten up all parts of the body in jerky movements, much as the walk of a tin-soldier.

Occasional stretching, tightening up of all bodily regions into a tight tremolo will bring blood consciously to the internal organs.

Slow exercising with small weights, 5 lb, 10., is excellent.

Effortless exercise, i.e. swinging of arms, legs

On the spot ball games are better than heavy hitting with a racket where capillaries of hand may become destroyed Thus golf, pingpong, catch, are excellent. Some handball is permissible.

Dancing with a partner is just about one of the best forms of exercising.

Stretch, then hold, as in Yoga. Breathe. Do it for all limbs.

Do not overexert yourself physically in extreme heat or icy cold temperatures.

CHAPTER XXIV

HOW TO ELIMINATE WITHOUT DIFFICULTY

Swing a ten lb weight slowly up, down and around.

Walk slowly on all fours; let body weight fall on palms of hands and soles of feet, either in push up position, bent over the bathtub or simply at the toilet seat. Shift body weight on all fours in a clockwise fashion, turning 5 lb. weight around in your hand.

Tighten abdominal region occasionally. Breathe deeply, pursing lips.

If necessary, introduce some softened, mild, perfumeless soap to induce a movement.

Hold a hot water bag. Massage legs slowly if necessary.

Drink some water during the process.

Light literature permissible but total darkness is best.

Much circulating air is important. Leave bathroom door open.

When stomach is full, push in the standing position.

When stomach is empty, you may need a potty to literally squeeze it out.

Always wait for a contraction for the final push.

Tighten up abodominal region.

In the standing position, shift body weight on all fours, push, supporting body on fingers placed on floor beside legs. It is important to press hands against some surface, bathtub, toilet seat, floor, etc.

Sit or walk around between evacuations.

Several evacuations are sometimes necessary.

Watch a cat eliminate and imitate.

Sometimes holding onto a bar is sufficient. Leaning head on hand may facilitate the process.

Complete silence is important.

When you have a growth in your rectum, hold on to a bar, shift body weight along hands and feet, very slowly, to induce contractions.

Never panic when blood appears in stools.

Sometimes pushing can temporarily rupture a tiny blood vessel. Because the lesion is internal, it will heal repidly.

Never operate a rectal tumor. Scar tissue on anal sphincter prevents normal expansion whereupon a colostomy becomes a necessity. Better learn to live with a tumor than undergo an operation.

CHAPTER XXV

HOW YOU CAN AVOID THE AGING PROCESS

Counterbalance an action by its opposing action: 3 meals, 3 bowel movements; 1 hour of standing, an hour seated; 1 hour of speaking, an hour of silence, etc.
Solitude and silence induce youthfulness, creativity and longevity.
Avoid exercise requiring the use of a heavy instrument to hit with.
Stay away from jobs requiring the continuous use of one's voice.
Stay away from jobs forcing constant expenditure of nervous tension, of energy of some kind. i.e. facing the public to sing, speak, etc.
Avoid the constant use of sereral large systems each day.
Balance the chills experienced with surges of heat in perspiration.
Avoid the sight of speeding trains.
Avoid excess bulk in diet.
Avoid several climaxes in succession.
Avoid forceful accomplishment of the sex act.
Practice moxibustion by allowing a stream of very hot water to remain for long periods on one spot of skin until a surge of heat is reached. Then move to another spot.
Sleep before 12 o'clock.
Get at least 7 hours of sleep each day.

CHAPTER XXVI

HOW TO OBTAIN THE BEST QUALITY OF SLEEP

Place two wool blankets above your mattress.
Sleep on a bed lined with several pillows or sleep above an eiderdown quilt for great relaxation.
Bundle yourself up for sound sleep in the winter.
Never sleep naked, even in hot summer months.
Sleeping on a couch with a high back is most relaxing.
Pillows behind your back when in bed, could have a similar effect.
Allow several hours between the last meal of the day and sleep.
Read some light literature before closing your eyes.
Tighten up your entire body very slowly into a tight shiver, before you fall asleep.
Do the same upon awakening. It may be called stretching with a yawn.
For sound sleep at night, do not expend excess energy in several directions during the day.
Dim lights and subdued sounds in the day are more conducive to deep sleep at night.
Make sure no bright lights or loud noises assail the sleeping person anytime.
When stomach is full, sleep with several pillows under your head.
When stomach is empty, sleep almost flat.
Don't be disturbed if you don't get your sleep some days. Simply do less work the next day and you will fall asleep.

Insomnia is always due to excess expenditure of energy in some direction. Enforced relaxation is necessary for all sorts of sleeplessness, from nervous   breakdowns to simple insomnia.

Deep sleep is externally shown when both arms are raised above head.

Peaceful sleep is assured when breathing is imperceptible.

Snoring, tossing and turning denotes restless sleep.

Light meals with careful preparation of foods can rid one of snoring.

Perspiration during sleep ensures continued health for a lifetime.

Keeping your head warm during sleep will prevent loss of hair for life.

Always keep windows open when you sleep, whether in warm weather or in the middle of winter.

Take the position of an L during sleep, if possible.

CHAPTER XXVII

HOW TO CHOOSE LIVING ORGANISMS USED
AS FOOD

Select foods from living organisms placed high on the scale of evolution: meats, fruits, fruit-like vegetables, flower-like vegetables.

An animal whose fat is edible is easier to digest than the opposite: pork, fowl are more digestible than lamb, beef.

Meat from a small animal is easier to digest than from an animal of 1,000 lbs.

When purchasing fish, large fish with scales and centrally located digestive tract are better than scaleless fish with a digestive system pushed to the side, i.e. striped bass versus blue-fish.

Large fish are more beneficial than tiny fish.

This holds true for animals without a backbone: large crabs, large shrimps, lobster, better than squid, tiny shrimps, etc.

Among fruits, the small fruits like grapes, are easier to digest than heavy skinned fruits like oranges, grapefruit.

The heaviest fruits are melons and tropical fruits.

Among vegetables, fruit-like vegetables, flower-like vegetables are better than shoots, stems and leaves.

Grain and seed are second to tomatoes, pepper, or fruit-like vegetables.

Heaviest vegetable are carrots, turnips, potatoes.

Lowest among vegetables are mushrooms and shoots.

Avoid skins of all organisms.

Avoid dark green, leafy vegetables.

Avoid internal organs as food: brains, tripe, kidneys, liver, tongue, heart.

Honey, a simple sugar, is better than cane sugar, a complex sugar.

Beans of all kinds are a source of complete proteins.

Light nuts like pistacchio nuts, are better than heavy nuts, i.e. almonds, Brazil nuts.

Learn to eat produce in season: Muscatel grapes in the fall, chestnuts in winter.

Try to obtain fruits from far away lands, whenever possible.

CHAPTER XXVIII

HOW TO SELECT FOODS IN GENERAL

Consume processed foods sparingly, i.e. ham, Swiss cheese, bologna, mortadella, pepperoni, salami, processed sausages.

Fresh foods are best.

Choose foods that rot fast when exposed to the air, milk, etc.

Avoid foods that take months to rot when placed on the table, i.e. breads, pastries, cookies.

In general foods that are on the liquid side are easier to digest than those that are dry, thick, greasy and heavy.

Avoid deep-fried foods.

Oily pastries are to be eaten sparingly.

Only some bread-like pastries like cheese Danish, can be eaten more often.

Some of the pies are among the most pleasant types of pastries.

Wine and liquor are to be sparingly intaken.

Saturated fats, i.e. pork fat, chicken fat, butter, better than unsaturated oils: corn oil, peanut oil, vegetable oil, crisco, etc. for your body makes is own unsaturated oils from saturated fats.

CHAPTER XXIX

HOW YOU CAN FORM A PERFECT HUMAN
BEING

Do not circumcise infant boys.

Breast feed as much and as long as possible.

If not, use a much diluted natural formula or dilute formula with a soup made of 2 level tablespoonfuls of corn starch and 1 quart of water.

Think about Mozart who was fed mostly water during the first year of life.

Do not administer vitamins in any form.

Only give diluted freshly squeezed juices as source of vitamin.

Let baby sleep as much as possible in a roomful of sunshine and fresh air.

Take him for long walks in a carriage where the shaking and rumble of wheels lulls him to deeper sleep.

Let him have his bottle ten years if he desires. Never force him to eat anything he doesn't wish to eat.

Never wake baby up for feedings. Let him tell you he's hungry. Whenever baby drools, lie him down.

Use little of bottled foods in supermarkets. You can make your own foods and either blend them or pass them in a mouli-baby.

Only after he has a mouthful of teeth should he be allowed to eat solid foods, and these must be cooked in small pieces.

If at any time the cartillages of the nose become pushed out of shape, dilute the formula or never give heavy foods.

CHAPTER XXX

HOW TO COOK FOODS FOR CONTINUED
HEALTH AND BEAUTY

Noiseless cooking is proper cooking.

In direct heat, cook over low heat, with constant stirring or almost constant watching(broiling). In indirect cooking, i.e. steaming, baking, medium heat should be used.

High heat used only for rending of fat, browning in deep fat.

Remove an item from heat as soon as its aroma is perceptible.

The color of vegetables should not change after cooking.

Never allow the smell of food to reek across the apartment.

Warm-up foods over medium high heat, with constant stirring.

When mixing foods, always cook each item separately until the point of smell, then combine together for a second or two.

Always undercook foods when they must be used in a recipe and cooked again.

Meat should be tenderized with the back of a butcher-knife if it is to be cooked in a large piece, i.e. pork chop, steak.

Better cut meats and vegetables up fine than use large pieces.

Always remove skins from vegetables, meats, fruits, before cooking.

When cooking a bird, always rend fat over high heat.

After fat is rent, sometimes bird is ready to be eaten.

A chopstick poked in will tell you if it is ready. Remove from heat.

Steamed foods and pot roasts are healthiest ways of cooking.

Halve the given amount of sugar in recipes for pies, cookies.

PART III

HOW TO BE AWARE OF ILLNESS

CHAPTER XXXI

HOW YOU CAN DIAGNOSE ILLNESSES

Throughout the ages it has been extremely difficult to pinpoint exactly the cause of an illness. With the viewpoint   of the body functioning in 6 systems, diagnosis of illness becomes a mere child's play, as you will see from the following.

Actually there are only 3 ways to choose from when it concerns causes of illnesses.

1. When the external appearance of a region or of the body changes, there is some anomaly in the food intake, i.e. either excess of one kind of food, late meals, too little fluids, too much starches, too much meat, too many vegetables, too little protein, heavy foods at night, etc.

Example. Robert D. had a particularly slow, cantankerous gait. When asked whether he was on a special diet, he revealed he only ate vegetables. This explained the reason for his cantankerous walk.

2. When internal regions of the body are affected, there has been excess activity in any of the remaining systems, i.e. too much sex, too much noise, excessive light, too much talking, singing, too many external stimuli, excessive standing, running.

Example: Gloria B. suffered from an ulcer in her stomach and stones in her kidney. She revealed that her job as a computer programmer exposed her to constant zooming noise all day long, 40 hours per week. The noise diverted so much blood away from her internal organs that all sorts of abnormal conditions developed.

3. When physical or chemical properties of the blood are affected, all remaining 5 systems must have their activities reduced, Thus in fever, liquids must comprise diet, lights must be dimmed down, no sounds should disturb the patient.

When physical and chemical properties are permanently disturbed,i.e. cancer, constant fever, diabetes, Addison's disease, a total change in lifestyle must be made. Thus early retirement becomes a necessity while silence, solitude and constant dieting are imperative.   When you diagnose illnesses, in general one must feel free both to ask and to answer questions. A series of questions on lifestyle, use of the 5 active systems, food habits, should rapidly enable you to pinpoint exactly, the cause of an illness and thereby prescribe a cure.

CHAPTER XXXII

THE SIGNIFICANCE OF EXTERNAL VITAL MANIFESTATIONS

Your breathing. The normal breathing rate is 8-25 per minute. Imperceptible breathing indicates freely flowing blood within blood vessels, with excellent digestion.

Impaired breathing with occasional gasping shows extremely slow blood flow with difficult digestion where mucous backs up nasal passages.

A change in diet, dim lights, solitude, relaxation, can improve the condition.

Your voice. Man's voice is a higher manifestation of life, thus a most strenuous feat. Your voice may be warm, highpitched, metallic, cold, resonant or other attributes. Your voice reflects how well your brain is irrigated, in turn indicating smooth functioning of the regulatory organs. When the quality of your voice changes, good sleep with much liquids become imperative.

Your posture. Upright posture is found in man alone. Upright posture indicates normal physical and chemical properties of the blood. Bent posture of varying degrees indicates degrees of removal from normal values, whether closer or farther from critical values. No posture signifies a state of coma. While a change of diet can improve a bent posture, fasting can help bring a patient out of a comatose state.

Your gait. Normal gait signifies optimum blood volume. When gait is serously impaired, there has been overtaxation in some vital activity.

Since time immemorial it is known that over indulgence in sex can result in hemiplegia, even quadriplegia. It is good to practice sex sparingly indeed.

Your hair and nails. Ever growing hair and nails indicate how well the blood is being regulated. Chipping nails with brittle hair that stays limp indicate poor regulation of body fluids, thus bad sleep. Fasting or partial fasting should improve the condition. Sometimes overexertion in some other vital activity can prevent optimum regulation at night. Relaxation should improve the condition.

Your skin. Your skin literally reflects the state of function of your endoctine glands. Velvety, smooth skin means optimum function of these glands of internal secretion. An ugly skin with blotches show overwork of glands. In general for constantly smooth skin, do not eat food by the pound or in large amounts.

Your eyes. These denote the state of your blood vessels. When eyes are almond-shaped, vessels are unclogged. The more haggard the eyes, the more clogged the blood vessels. A period of fasting should improve the condtion. The size of your eyes denote how careful you are in all your undertaking. Huge eyes show reckless overall behavior, while small eyes denote extreme carefulness in life.

Your eyelids. When kidneys are overworked, your eyelids will become swollen and puffed up. Heavy eyelids denote extreme restlessness of body tissues. Eyelids with the internal epicanthic fold denotes peacefullness in all vital functions.

Your cheeks. Full cheeks indicate the constancy of your blood volume. When cheeks are hollow, blood volume is seriously overtaxed from some excessive physical or other exertion. Plenty of liquids and slowing down of vital functions can restore full cheeks.

Your lips. These indicate whether you are generally relaxed or subjected to extreme nervous tension. Those whose lips disappear should not undertake any sort of public activity where extreme nervous tension assails them. In general full lips indicate great sensuality.

Your ears. Strangely enough, your ears are extremely significant. They actually show whether you will live long or not. In general large ears denote longevity while tiny ears are a definite sign of a much shorter life. However if an individual with large ears uses up his vital functions in excess, he will yet live a shortened life. Ears that seem detached from the head indicate carelessness and slovenliness in general. On the contrary ears that stick to the head denote extreme carefulness and an overall peaceful life.

Hairiness. Hair on the skin is simply nature's means to provide more heat to the body during the time of growth. Restless sleep with heavy breathing promote the growth of hair in adolescence. More careful preparation of foods can prevent excessive growth of hair in childhood.

Your breathing and your pulse rate. Taken together, breathing and pulse rate indicate the total blood volume through the entire regulatory organs: heart, lungs, kidneys, skin, endocrine glands. Thus 2 beats to 1 inhalation signifies optimum blood wolume. 3 beats to 1 inhalation shows considerably reduced flow. 4 beats to 1 inhalation indicates approaching death. These values are to be taken only upon awakening. Only partial fasting can help improve the condition. Otherwise a dilute liquid diet becomes imperative.

Your urine. Everyone is aware that the yellow color of urine means that poisons are continuously leaving the body. Sometimes the urine may appear white. Extreme nervous tension coupled with overexertion in any of the 5 active organ-systems can bring on such a condition. Enforced relaxation or complete inactivity will soon restore the condition to normal. If the condition persists a liquid diet becomes imperative.

Your feces. The color, smell and consistency of daily feces are important indicators of health. When extra soft there has been intake of some concentrated drug or food When black with a sickly, fermented smell, fermentation is taking place within the rectum and poisonous materials are being reabsorbed within the blood stream. One must never be panic-striken when changes occur to feces While they are normally brown and pasty with a distinctive smell, the most important thing is daily elimination. Even in a most terminal condition daily elimination can delay death with certainty.

Your breath. Everyone knows how sweet a baby's breath can be. Our breath literally shows how well your digestion is going on. A sweet breath shows good digestion while a literally foul breath means you are close to the end of your life. Your breath can well indicate whether you are in a terminal state or not, so be wary of it.

Your general bodily shape. Shape of body is an index of health. A slender waistline indicates good, rapid digestion. It is usually associated with abundant hair on the head. The opposite is also true.

If you are born with a defect. People usually will shy away from a birth defect. Actually a birth defect is simply nature's automatic means of arresting activity in the defective region in order to preserve the organism with a full lifespan. Thus a retarded child is not supposed to exert himself mentally. He should simply be allowed to live and enjoy himself in his simple way as long as possible. A person born without limbs is truly not supposed to work with his hands so that he may live as long as possible. And so on. I came to the above conclusion simply by reasoning that work requires motion of blood to capillaries of the active region. When the region is not present or defective, blood cannot flow to the area, in turn preserving the motor from a great depletion.

This kind of reasoning should make a defective person much more acceptable to society.

Your hair and nails. These constantly growing parts of your body indicate how well regulation is taking place. Broken nails that chip, brittle hair that falls eaily indicate poor regulation of body fluids. A well-balanced diet coupled with careful mastication can preserve glossy hair with strong nails. Relaxation, long hours of sleep can prevent hair form falling limp.

Hiccuping, sneezing, wheezing, coughing. You will note that in every instance, breathing is affected. Actually they indicate overactivity in one of the 5 organ-systems. Relaxation, warm clothing, a light diet can arrest these disturbing symptoms.

Silence and solitude waive these conditions altogether.

Your blood. Healthy blood is a deep red color. Your menstrual flow should show you the condition of your blood. If it is very dark, it may be overloaded with poisons. A period of fasting is beneficial. If your blood appears pink and floats, remove all starches from your diet. You may have abundant white cells in which case constant dieting becomes imperative.

CHAPTER XXXIII

SOME MEDICAL MYTHS

High Blood Pressure. Today high blood pressure is always treated by prescribing a salt free diet. This is dangerous as blood is truly salty in taste. Without salt our blood can stop flowing properly.

Actually any overexertion causes high blood pressure, i.e. during sex, when we get up, after a big meal, after physical exertion, etc. Greater awareness in all our vital activities can prevent a rise in blood pressure.

Anemia. Usually a test for anemia is always done on blood from a finger prick or from the vein in the arm, thus an extremity of the body. For this reason a blood test cannot be trusted, for after a big meal, during pregnancy, after physical exertion, etc., blood has been diverted away from the extremities to sustain the above vital functions. At this point any blood test taken would show anemia. For this reason one should never trust a hospital test for anemia.

For a truly worthwhile test one should be allowed to lie down an entire half hour before the test.

Many diets today are prescribed according to blood pressure test and blood count tests. One must be wary of such advice. You should always analyze yourself and see in what direction you have overexerted yourself. Once the cause is found, its removal will restore your condition to normal. Personally I would never trust either of the above tests.

CHAPTER XXXIV

HOW YOU CAN COPE WITH PAIN

Up to the present pain has remained an unsolvable mystery. Actually there are two types of pain, local pain and systemic pain.

Local pain affects small capillary areas while systemic pain involves large capillary areas.

Local pain: you experience local pain when something enters your body, when something acts on your body or when you do work.

When something enters your body and desires to leave:

Bullets, tar in gums; in every case capillaries are affected. Because no more blood can be diverted to the region, pain is felt. Once removed, blood flow is restored and pain disappears.

When something acts on your body:

Holding a package. Normally there is no pain. At a point when package becomes too heavy and you must lay it down, immediate removal of package restores normal blood flow. If package is not lain down, all your hand capillaries may break and your hand may become impotent for life.

When something acts on your body:

A slight touch gives an itchy sensation. When pushed further you will feel pressure until pain is experienced. It is again a result of capillary distention.When pain becomes unbearable the pressure must be removed immediately otherwise all capillaries may break.

Some other types of local pain:

Bruises: When something acts on the body suddenly and heavily, you will experience a bruise. This must immediately be rubbed until pain disappears otherwise under conditions of slow blood flow, a tumor may develop.

Needle-like pains: abnormal regeneration of body cells may result in needle-like pain. Because body fluids are involved, removal of all processed foods, alcohol, heavy greasy foods, excess sugar from the diet is most important .

We all know that body cells slough off and die during a lifetime. Only optimum environment of body fluids ensures normal regeneration of cells without pain.

Pain in joints: Joints present a knot to the circulation. For this reason deposits of excess absorbed nutrients may develop at joints. Partial fasting with a liquid diet will soon restore the condition to normal. It is a good idea to be comfortably clothed from head to toe and never expose any part of your body to the air.

Systemic pain: When large capillary regions are involved in pain, we have systemic pain in the area.

A sleeping limb: while a sleeping limb may not cause pain as such, you will notice that if you were to use it suddenly unawares, terrible pain may result. You must always allow circulation to restore itself before you use a sleeping limb. Sudden exertion of such a limb may break all capillaries of the area.

Headaches: because of its 2 quart size, pain in the head is a serrous systemic pain. Temporarily remove a headache by tightening up the head region into a tight shiver while pursing lips and intaking a deep breath. Hold, then relax. For permanent relief, sleep soundly or induce a complete bowel elimination.

Headaches are always caused by overexertion in one of the 5 active systems. It is best to avoid large chunks of meat, heavy foods, if headaches become frequent. If they last 12 hours or more, you should retire permanently.

Childbirth pains: A full uterus represents a large system indeed and much blood is lost after the baby is born It is important to drink much water during labor. Place legs up against wall during contractions. Especially during the final push you should freely be given water otherwise terrible consequences may result(blood shot eyes, even death, forceps baby). You can reduce child-birth pains by placing your legs up against the wall during labor.

Other types of systemic pain are the loss of a limb or limbs, toothaches, especially when serveral teeth are involved. Those who suffer much systemic pain must lead a quiet life, far from commitments. Silence and a peaceful life induce longevity for those that are weak.

In general, all pain is caused by a lack of blood flow to the region. Either rubbing, removal of foreign material either within the region or from another region, will restore normal blood flow and remove pain.

Pain experienced in surgery.

It is the custom in China to practice surgery with acupuncture. Over the centuries the Chinese have found that one can cut open an area and work on internal organs without the patient feeling pain.

Pain is transmitted by the myelin sheath surrounding nerve fibers. My research shows that all nerve fibers supplying internal organs are non-myelinated, thus unable to transmit the sensation of pain. The Chinese instinctively knew through practice, assuring themselves that this was true. The needle placed either nearby within a muscle, or far away, simply served to divert blood away from the spot undergoing operation, to prevent excessive bleeding in the wound and raise the pain threshold.

For those who fear an operation without anesthesia, it is safe to receive simply a local anesthesia to dullen pain within muscles. Our internal organs only perceive some dull pain, a pull or a prick, never extreme pain.

CHAPTER XXXV

HOW TO COPE WITH YOUR TEETH

Cavities: do not get a filling made unless the cavity gives you a chill whenever you use the tooth at meals. A cavity in a deciduous tooth can be waived as the tooth will be lost anyway. However have a filling done if discomfort is felt.

Pyorrhea: an initial treatment from a dental surgeon is a must. If condition persists, get yourself a scaler*. From time to time, use your finger to feel around the gums of your teeth. If there is a slight itchy sensation, use a scaler like your dental surgeon and gently scrape the tar out. Some bleeding will accompany scraping.

The bleeding will stop after the tar is removed.

Toothache: continued treatments as above indicated should avoid toothaches for life. However, if toothaches should happen, insert the scaler during a painful contraction and scrape and scrape. After bleeding stops, your tooth will be saved. Extraction of a tooth becomes necessary only if a tooth is very loose, never otherwise.

Pyorrhea is caused by acid from digestion of foods, backing up the tract, gnawing at roots of teeth. For this reason heavy foods should be avoided by those prone to pyorrhea. Follow advice given in chapter on digestion, to waive pyorrhea for life.

---

* a scaler in the shape of a broken half moon is best. They cost around $5.00 at any dental supply store.

CHAPTER XXXVI

SOME ENIGMATIC ILLNESSES EXPLAINED

Epilepsy: the 'Sacred Disease' of the past best shows that the living body works in 3 large active organ-systems: the digestive system, the muscles and bones and the regulatory organs. An analysis of a Grand Mal Seizure shows this to be true. The patient falls to the ground, losing all voluntary control(muscles and bones inactive) foam oozes from the mouth(digestion has stopped), the body stiffens to a tight tremolo(automatic activity of the sympathetic nervous system forcing blood within the entire regulatory organs). Actually the patient fell asleep unawares. Epilepsy is a condition showing the poor automatic function of the sympathetic nervous ganglia, the result of poor sleep during the first year of life when automaticity of the autonomic nervous system is established.

To combat seizures, the patient should wilfully tighten up his body as many times as necessary during the day. It should waive the need of automatic seizures. Also, a light diet should always be observed, thus providing the sympathetic nervous division with an optimum supply of blood.

Parkinson's: characterized by stooped posture, slow movement, fixity of facial expression and tremor of hands. There is tendency to lose balance and fall. Yet in the completely relaxed position no tremor is manifested. In general the greater the conscious effort, the greater the tremor.

This illness shows disturbance in the appearance of the body, thus some anomaly in the food intake. In this case too few liquids. Actually Parkinson's indicates a much diminished blood volume, sufficient only to fill the entire regulatory organs in the relaxed state. As soon as the patient is required to perform conscious activity (where blood volume must flow to muscles and bones). tremor is manifested. Tremor becomes very marked when voluntary activity is done.

Increasing the intake of liquids should improve the condition rapidly. In general a quiet life, far from commitments should be the trend.

Cancer: The scourge of mankind for centuries, cancer is still much dreaded in the XXth Century.

Cancer can afflict people of all ages. It can be triggered by excess activity in any one of the 5 active organ-systems, while fear, sadness, fright, constant hurrying can rapidly stir its oncoming. Usually eating beyond satiation can bring on cancer very rapidly. a lump felt in the throat when swallowing shows its beginning. With the lack of hunger pains, one still must eat. At that point any bruise or burn can trigger a tumorous formation.

Tumors form because our body cells die and are constantly replaced. When in a normal internal medium, body cells will regenerate normally, but when your blood flow slows down, the changed environment will cause abnormal regeneration.

Our internal environment is a product of the foods ingested. Most all foods turn into sugar which in turn forms alcohol. When a molecule of water is removed between 2 alcohols, you will have the formation of ether, under high body temperatures. When your body is bathed in an environment of ether, abnormal cellular regeneration will take place.

The above explanation alllows us to help ourselves when we are afflicted   with cancer. Those foods able to produce much ether, are to be avoided. Thus fats, alcohol, complex sugars, sweet pastries, breads, most all dry starches. In fact only some protein in the form of meat, cheese, milk, where the fat is dilute, are permissible, while vegetables and fruits are   equally safe.   Wet starches like pasta, wheat starch dough, dough made of boiling water should be the only starches permissible. Of course rice made into a watery softness is equally permissible.

In cancer, daily elimination presents a great problem. Most bodily functions become so slow that nothing seems to be able to descend the tract. Enforced relaxation is a must, while warm clothing must be adopted. Early retirement is a must while solitude and peacefulness can yet allow a few years of life. Tension, fear, great sadness, even sex, are to be avoided, for otherwise one can easily reach a terminal state.

When foods become poison to the system, they are to be treated as such. Licking, sucking, picking at foods will facilitate daily functions. One can yet live a good 20 years with cancer.

Today breast tumors often develop. It is important to learn to squeeze out all milk from breasts during several months after childbirth. This will prevent tumorous growths in later life.

In general, always rub a bruise immediately to avoid growth of tumors.

PART IV

SOME SUGGESTIONS FOR TERMINAL STATES

SOME SUGGESTIONS FOR PERMANENT STATES

CHAPTER XXXVII

SIGNS WARNING OF AN APPROACHING
TERMINAL STATE.

Vague hunger pains.
A trickling sensation in legs.
Extreme cold in legs.
Almost constant chills.
Nails that chip easily.
Incessant activity with the inability to relax.
Lengthy headaches.
Constant slight fever.
A haggard look.
Ease of infection.
Extremely difficult elimination.
Three to four heart beats per inhalation upon
awakening.
Fermented smell of feces.
Frequently colorless urine.
Ringing in the head.
Needle-like pain here and there.

CHAPTER XXXVIII

SIGNS OF A TERMINAL CONDITION

Extreme foul breath.
Teeth that literally rot away.
Constant pain in kidneys or liver.
Difficult breathing, with gasping.
Extreme cold.
Rapid build-up of wax in ears, causing stinging pain.
Inability to bear loud noise and strong light.
No hunger pain yet desire to eat.
Great difficulty with daily elimination.
Fever.
Heavy pulse.
Putrid smell of feces.
Strong body odor.
The feeling that nothing works in your body any longer.
Lengthy ringing in the head.
A dark, earthy colored complexion.
Caving-in of the temporal region of your head.

CHAPTER XXXIX

HOW TO COPE WITH A TERMINAL STATE

You must resign yourself to constant dieting.
Bundle yourself up for sleep: bonnet, wool sweater, leggings, etc. Complete silence, solitude, induce smooth body function.
Dilute proteins, fruits, beneficial.
Starches are to be intaken sparingly indeed. Only some light starch like soft rice, wheat starch, corn starch should be used. Dry breads, cakes, cookies, fried foods are to be avoided like poison.
Pick solids in tiny bits. Lick or suck foods, treat foods like poison Avoid hospital tests at all costs: ligating, poking, pricking, X rays, blood tests, injections, drugs, operations.
Long wool skirts, wool pants, turtle neck shirts and sweaters a must.
Long cotton dresses in summer to induce perspiration.
Avoid excitement of all kinds. Become a solitary recluse.
An even disposition is important.
Beware of great joy or extreme sadness.
Early retirement a must.
Avoid sex.
A liquid diet or semi-liquid diet becomes a must.
Remove wax from ears by using vaseline to soften up the wax. Eliminate at least twice daily.

Both abundant wax in ears and abundant feces in rectum can cause convulsions. It is important to remove them daily from your body.

Your blood literally becomes like that of a cat. Like the big cats, a protein diet with fruits is all that is permissible. You may still live 9 years more, like a cat.

Be aware of pain and tighten up a painful region to a tight tremolo whenever you perceive it.

CHAPTER XL

WHEN YOU WILL UNDERTAKE A FAST

When you feel sudden, terrific pain in your legs, feet, head or other extremity, or stinging pain in your heart.

When your body swells, a sign of kidney failure, meaning the kidneys have burst and poisons are pouring into your body cavity.

When you can no longer breathe normally and must gasp constantly.

When your heart beats heavily 4 or 5 beats to an inhalation upon awakening.

When you have extreme difficulty walking or mounting steps.

When you know the end is near at hand.

When you feel you are about to experience convulsions.

When you begin to fear death.

When you feel bursting of your wind pipe.

When sleep can be obtained only if your head is propped up with a pile of pillows.

When you feel constant pain in the lower regions of your body.

CHAPTER XLI

WHAT FASTING CAN DO FOR YOU

It will force an entire system into inactivity.

It will force blood flow within body cells and blood vessels, prevent further build-up of deposits and permit poisons to be eliminated from the blood stream.

It will bring back hunger pains.

Your urine will be very yellow with eliminated poisons.

It will rejuvenate your body.

It will allow your regulatory organs to work to the utmost to combat foreign bacteria, as white blood cells will rapidly engulf them and prevent their further proliferation.

It will bring you back to life when in a terminal state.

It will make you sexy.

CHAPTER XLII

SOME FASTING TECHNIQUES

Approach fasting slowly by gradual elimination of foods.

A diet of pasta mixed with cheeses, meats is a good way to begin to eliminate foods. These must be gradually eliminated. Eventually a diet of some hot cafe-au-lait and grapes or orange juice can be adopted for the rest of times.

Suck juices of oranges, grapes, discarding skin and pits.

Freshly squeezed juices may be intaken up to 2 or 3 quarts, safely, per day.

For quick results, juices taken in the morning, hot water or tea for the remaining hours of the day, kept up until hunger returns. Body must be kept extremely warm during a fast.

Enforce at least 1 bowel movement a day.

Use the aroma of delicious but oily foods to satisfy your central nervous system during a fast. Always smell it until satiation, A jar of peanut butter is excellent.

Wear mocassins to promote fullness and ease up a fast Completely flat shoes give a feeling of intense satisfaction. Take as many days to return to a normal diet as it took you to achieve a fast.

Break the fast carefully as you can experience a foecal impaction and will be unable to eliminate for a month.

If you cannot fast completely, simply adopt a dilute liquid diet of light soups, cafe-au lait and juices, for the remaining years of your life.

Sieve dilute, clear broth and diluted fruit juice for an ultimate diet.

CHAPTER XLIII

HOW TO DEAL WITH VIRULENT
BACTERIAL INFECTIONS

Leprosy, Syphilis and Tuberculosis are known as virulent bacterical infections. It is common knowledge today that these illnesses can be eradicated when they are detected in the early stages. Antibiotics can dispose of virulent bacteria in no time. However, if they are not discovered until much later, they become seemingly incurable.

In such instances, it becomes necessary to instill fear in the patient. Only fear will induce him to undertake a lengthy fast, the only cure for these sadly afflicted people.

It is important to know that when you are affected with syphilis and are in a latent stage, you are actually in a terminal state and the next organ to be affected will be nervous tissue. When this happens, there will be total loss of voluntary activity, sleep will not occur, no body function will take place properly. It is said that hospitals today are redundant with advanced cases of syphilis.

I have personally cured a case where a young girl suffered from syphilis for five years No antibiotic had an effect upon her condition and try as she may, nothing helped. I placed her on a juice diet. For 13 full days she drank and ate nothing else but juices. After the 13 day ordeal, her breath became sweet and her boyfriend married her.

In leprosy, it is common knowledge today that parts of the body will simply drop off and death will ensue. While I have not had the occasion to cure an advanced case of leprosy, I have cured a woman in the beginning stages of the disease.

Seven days of juice fasting did the trick. After that the germ never returned again.

In general those who suffer from leprosy should not eat starches. The only kind of starch permissible is a little pasta or a dough made with wheat starch. The saying that the more ill you are the more careful the preparation of food must be, is true to the letter. Delicious foods prepared with extreme care should be the habit.

In tuberculosis once all lung tissue has been invaded by the bacteria, there will be total inability to oxygenate body tissues. At that point death will ensue.

Though I have never met with a case of tuberculosis, I believe a juice fast should cure it in no time at all. In general sex should be avoided by those afflicted with a terminal illness. Sex makes it more difficult to effect the cure.

Total rest, relaxation should be the trend for all these conditions.

Those who are weak and prone to leprosy and tuberculosis must be aware of the functions of the 5 active organ-systems.

No overexertion should be the rule during the remainder of one's life.

CHAPTER XLIV

WHAT YOU CAN DO IN AN EMERGENCY

Today, it is appalling how frantic people become when someone faints or becomes suddenly unconscious. Usually one calls the ambulance and the patient is rushed to the hospital where the attending physician orders an injection. If the patient is lucky, he will survive the injection, otherwise he succumbs immediately.

Let us analyze the unconscious state. The patient is unable to assume upright posture, indicating abnormal properties of the blood. If he gasps for breath, extremely reduced blood volume is indicated. The sudden introduction of an injection can greatly diminish further the blood volume through the regulatory organs and death may immediately ensue.

From the above, it is clear that modern methods of handling emergencies are truly not very efficient. Let us see how they can be improved.

An unconscious person is completely shut off from the world of sights and sounds, however the millions of tiny sense organs on the surface of the skin are present, waiting to be exploited Receptor organs of the skin are terminals of the sensory nerves. When they are stimulated, three types of structures are excited; smooth muscle (blood vessels), gland and skeletal muscle.

Throughout the centuries mankind has practiced massage. Massage renews vitality of nerves and spinal cord, increases secretion of glands of digestive tract, aids digestion and assimilation. Today, medical science is aware that warm stimulations of the skin produce a reaction in blood vessels and increases body temperature as a whole. This in turn increases circulation through muscles and bones, restoring proper respiration and digestion, glandular secretion or excretions.

Due to the greatly diminished blood volume within the regulatory organs of an uncouscious person, massage must be practiced with extreme care. To begin with, effleurage or gentle stroking of the skin should be the trend. Gently stroke the head, neck and chest regions of the patient who must remain fully clothed. When respiration is normally restored, massage a little stronger by friction. Slow friction helps interchange of tissue fluids.

When finally the patient is conscious, present him with a glass of warm water and continue with the massage. Only when full consciousness is restored can you use all other forms of massage which includes clapping, hacking, beating and pounding. The patient will tell you when to stop or you can judge for yourself. At any event massage should not be prolonged unnecessarily due to the weakened state of the patient.

PART V

SOME MEDICAL MYSTERIES SOLVED

CHAPTER XLV

HOW YOU CAN UNDERSTAND YOUR SLEEP MECHANISM

Since time immemorial man has been intrigued by the mechanism of sleep. One of the main reasons why it has been so difficult to solve the problem is simply due to the fact that man's body is not transparent. In some lower transparent organisms, the snake, the butterfly, where the thinness of the skin allows a view of the interior of the body, the following patterns have been observed, both at rest, at work and during sleep.

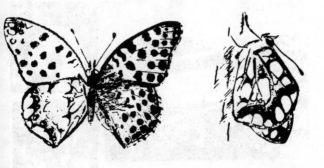

Fig. 5 The pearly butterfly pinned up to show the right side and the left underside(After Portmann)

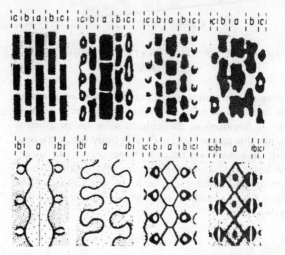

Fig. 6 Pattern variation in Python. A single specimen may have a number of these patterns in different regions of its body(After Portmann)

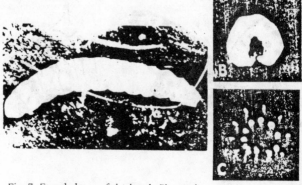

Fig. 7 Female larva of the beetle Phengodes.
A. Dorsal view. B. lateral view. C. luminous specimen in dark (After Prosser and Brown.)

Thus if our body were transparent, we would also be able to see a similar pattern at work and during sleep.

Actually sleep involves the regulatory organs innervated by the sympathetic nervous system. The latter allows blood to automatically fill up the large body of organs which comprise the entire regulatory organs: the heart, lungs, kidneys, skin, and endocrine glands. Because you need to have a heart of some sort before a brain of any kind can be developed, these organs are therefore closely tied.

You will notice that when you read some light literature before going to sleep, actually you are bringing blood to your brain. The next organ to receive blood will be the heart and of course the other regulatory organs.

You can imagine how much blood must fill up the entire set of regulatory organs. For this reason whenever your body relaxes, either seated or lying down, when all other stimuli are toned down, you will rapidly fall asllep.

Light sleep involves slight overfilling of the regulatory organs whild deep sleep signifies optimum overfilling of same.If there is any kind of activity going on within your body such as digestion or if your rectum is filled, you will not be able to fall asleep as readily. Removal of these disturbances will restore sleep.

The amount of work done during the day by the 5 active systms can also affect the volume of blood available at night to fill up the large body of organs. For this reason it is not a good idea to overexert yourself in any direction during the waking hours.

While the mechanism of sleep is not difficult to visualize, more important yet is the function of sleep. Actually sleep regulates the physical and chemical properties of the blood, restoring back to normal values, any deviation incurred during the day. This shows how important sleep is.

If for some reason you cannot sleep an adequate amount for one night, there is no need to worry. Simply analyze yourself and make sure you do not expend your energies in too many directions the following day. Serious consequences can arise if you do not follow this advice.

NERVOUS BREAKDOWNS

Up to the present nervous breakdowns are some of the most feared disturbances. This simply because the mechanism and function of sleep have not been understood. Now that I have explained it, it is easy to see that any excessive activity by the 5 active organ systems can cause a nervous breakdown, particularly activity of a voluntary kind: mental work, physical exertion, sex. In other words too much blood destroyed by work as cells rush through capillaries, diminishes the blood volume to such an extent that at night blood can no longer fill up the large body of regulatory organs.

While people suffering from a nervous breakdown have been interned in hopitals sometimes for years, even with eventual loss of their mind, there is truly only one simple solution to the problem. Because voluntary activity caused the disturbance, voluntary relaxation will restore sleep. For this reason you must enforce total body relaxation in order to restore the lost volume of blood and bring sleep back to normal.

CHAPTER XLVI

HOW YOU CAN UNDERSTAND LIFE AND DEATH

LIFE:

Everywhere around us we have ample occasion to notice life, yet until the present it has been impossible to explain it precisely in words.

Actually life can be explained in terms of the motion of blood to active capillaries. Thus whenever you pick something up in your hand, when you speak, listen, walk, etc., a flow of blood moves to the opened capillaries of the region, resulting in the respective vital manifestation: speech, hearing, walking, etc.

This explanation allows us to understand the cause for withered limbs. The sadly afflicted limb truly cannot wilfully divert a greater flow of blood to the capillaries because the nerves are non-functional. Thus enough blood flows through them to maintain a deathlike sort of life without movement.

The constant motion of blood to capillaries, i.e. life, is possible only because blood is regulated within normal physical and chemical values, thus at night during sleep. For this reason it is important to sleep before midnight after which air temperature lowers, Sleeping under lowered tempertures will affect your own body temperature.

Because blood can be regulated within three range of limits, we can say there are three types of vital manifestations. When blood is regulated within normal limits you will have normal activity. When blood is regulated within critical values, you will have erroneous vital activity. When blood properties are regulated within lethal limits, you will be in a state of coma.

DEATH:

Similar to life, we have had ample occasion to notice death, yet strangely enough no one has yet been able to define or visualize it exactly.

As we move down the scale of evolution, you will notice that in lower organisms there is much less vital manifestation. Lower organisms have regulatory organs that are extremely primitive and under-developed.

Because of the above, death can be explained as a waning of the regulatory organs, the inability to maintain proper regulation of physical and chemical properties of the blood.

The continuous action of your heart ties all parts together. When one of the large artery bursts or when extreme pain in extremities bursts blood vessels, death will ensue.

While death can be extremely painful in adolescence, actually death should not be as painful in old age. Suicides show us how great the pain experienced must be before we can kill ourselves They either involve jumping off a great height, being run over by a train, electrocution, dismemberment or the like.

Approaching death is usually warned by continuous headaches, for pain in the head indicates that the next organ to be affected will be the heart, for living organisms must have a heart of some kind before a brain of any sort can be developed. Headaches warn us that we must stop further damaging activities, especially those involving large capillary surfaces: physical exertion, sex, excess food.

Today many jobs present real hazards to health. Most of these require exertion of one's voice before a public: university professors, operatic singing, etc. While reducing the size of classrooms and using loudspeakers during a lecture can help save one's energy, it is especially important to use several singers in operatic performance. If we can accept any singer to take the part of Alfredo in La Traviata, we should then be able to accept several Alfredos during one performance. Not only more jobs would be made available to singers but it will most certainly save a singer's energy and prolong his lifespan.

It is time to realize that our lifespan does not exceed 75 years. We must learn to relax and enjoy the accumulated wealth instead of using all our energy to seemingly earn money which we can barely use.

Many conditions in modern cities can contribute to a shortened life. Such are the constant loud rumbling of cars wherever a beautiful avenue is found. I believe that if cars were forced to run at 10 miles per hour within city limits, city dwellers would begin to have a more peaceful life.

While skyscrapers hide the sun from so many, it has also been the cause of crime, for huge things cause fear, in turn inducing meanness to result in crime. It is time to do away with these structures and live close to the earth as in the Orient.

Not only massive and tall building cause crime, but they are extremely tiresome to the body. This may be the greatest cause for the many cases of premature aging found in the western world. Buildings should be made to fit the size of a human being. Buildings should not be constructed for the whole of humanity. It is time to consider human beings as individuals, not as masses of cattle.

The last issue concerns the seasons. The animal kingdom has shown us for centuries that life begins in the springtime, yet time and again schools, artistic endeavours begin their seasons in the fall. We must always observe the animals for they have greater instinct than we do. Mankind should start to think about beginning seasons towards the springtime. This would allow little children to sleep more during winter months when the air temperature is much lowered.

CHAPTER XLVII

HOW YOU CAN UNDERSTAND
THE AGING MECHANISM

Similar to sleep, the invisible aging process has stirred writers over the centuries to compile many volumes of research. Because aging is an invisible force, threefold in character, it has been extremely difficult to pinpoint exactly, its mechanism.

The threefold character of aging specifically deals with the capillaries, Pascal's principle, and the regulatory organs,

1. The breaking of capillary walls.

I explained in Part 1 how capillary walls can break. Thus forceful action of any kind causes blood cells to flow within capillaries in large clumps, forcing their way within the tiny vessels, tearing some of them into a million bits.

When many capillaries are torn, the metabolism of the region will be diminished and poisons will begin to stack up, changing the appearance of the area. You must make sure you do not forcefully perform your vital activities during a lifetime, simply to maintain viable capillaries. You can also keep in mind that you only have so many capillaries in any region. Once torn they can never be restored.

2. The action of depletion of blood within a set of organs.

In Part 1 I explained how activity within a system depletes all other regions, the sum of the depletions being equal to the quantity flowing through the one active region.

When a region is depleted of blood, circulation lessens to the region and poisons will begin to accumulate. It will change the appearance of the organ and with time, of the whole body. For this reason it is good to analyze your vital functions daily and make sure that you do not forcefully exert several large organ-systems at once.

3. The combined action of the two previous processes eventually react upon the regulatory organs which receive a great supply of blood only during sleep. Only smooth functioning of the regulatory organs will enable life to continue indefinitely. For this reason you must be watchful and make sure that not too many large capillary areas are being overtaxed during a lifetime. By large capillary areas. I mean the exertion of your voice for loud singing, the sex act, mental work, deafening noise and blinding lights continuously, excess food. Even continuous pregnancies represent the abuse of a definitely large capillary surface.

The abuse of several large capillary surfaces can cause your body to shrink.

One of the best ways to preserve yourself is total isolation into complete silence and semi-darkness, once in a while. This allows your body to restore itself.

While the threefold effect of aging is the greatest force, the next most important factor is the way fire is used to cook foods. The proper rebuilding of all parts of the body depends upon the quality of nutrients. When foods are overcooked, the vitamin content is lost while the bonds tying atoms and molecules fall apart.

They will not provide the proper nutrients to rebuild body tissue. As a result the body will become flabby and age. Proper use of fire will preserve vitamins and minerals and provide excellent tools to properly rebuild tissues and cells and give them a firm appearance.

CHAPTER XLVIII

THE CAUSE OF EVOLUTION

Last century Charles Darwin's Origin of Species received universal acclaim for his concept of natural selection with the survival of the fittest as the evolutionary force throguhout the ages.

Since his time many other theories of evolution have been propounded, none of which are conclusive. They have opened up new fields of interest yet at the same time have created more problems in terms of evolution.

In 1969 I developed a hypothesis, using the trends and forces of evolution to prove my point of view. I showed that evolution is a slow change resulting in a gradual but definite narrowing of the physical and chemical properties of the blood, to reach its peak narrowness in man.

This gradual but constant decrease in variability assumes the picture of a triangle, as follows:

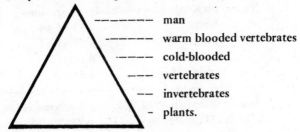

```
——————  man
—————  warm blooded vertebrates
————  cold-blooded
———  vertebrates
——  invertebrates
—  plants.
```

To show how this occurs, here are the normal blood sugar content of a few species of animals:

TABLE I

Normal Variation of Blood Sugar Content
per 100 cc of blood

Man	80 -120 mg
Ducks	100-160 mg
Chickens	200-250 mg
Scup	15.3 - 116.3 mg
Goose fish	0 - 10 mg

Source: Barcroft, 1934, p.78. For Man,
I.J. Routh, "Fundamentals of Inorganic, Organic and
Biological Chemistry", P. 397.

Again the ph of the blood follows a similar pattern

TABLE II

Normal ph Range of a few kinds of organisms

Man	7.33 - 7.44
Frogs	6.32 - 7.13
Insects	6.4-8.0
Invertebrates	3.5 - 8.3

Source: Barcroft, 1934, p.4. For invertebrates,
Kudo, "Protozoology," 1954, p.25, 26, 27.

While properties of the blood became narrower,
the brain on the contrary, became larger, reaching its
peak development in man.

At the same time the facial angle became straighter while the posture changed from a horizontal posture to a curved posture, raising mouthparts from ground level to man's upright posture.

As these external changes took place, internal upheavals occurred. From unicellular amoebae immersed in a liquid medium, multicellular animals developed, divided into invertebrates and vertebrates.

With the development of external characteristics, internal anatomical and physiogical changes simultaneously took place.

From a complete absence of regulatory organs in plants, the presence of a heart beomes visible in inverterebrates where valves propel the blood circulating within the body. A tubular heart may be found in earthworms, the two-chambered heart in fishes, the three-chambered heart in frogs and finally the four-chambered heart in warm blooded birds and mammals. The presence of a heart gradually enabled better separation of arterial and venous blood, in turn an increasingly more complex nervous system developed. One must have a heart of some sort before a brain of any kind can be developed.

From sensory cells in lowly animals, we see the presence of tiny ganglia in insects, earthworms. In frogs and birds the brain is pea-sized, to become highly convoluted in the brain of mammals and of course man, whose highly developed nervous system

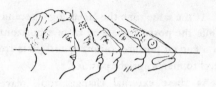

Fig. 8 . The evolution of the facial angle. (After Witowski).

enabled its separation into three great divisions, namely the brain, the sympathetic ganglia and the parasympathetic ganglia, all three divisions tied together by the spinal cord.

The division of labor within the nervous system enabled the three nerve centers to control the capillaries of the six systems, providing better direction in the growth of bodily parts: perfect regulatory organs, internal fertilization and development of embryo, as compared to external fertilization and development of the young: three dimensional vision as compared to forward vision; internal skeleton with muscle attachments as compared to external skeleton; sex organs to be aroused at will instead of fornication and heat in lower animals, etc.

The improvement of anatomical structures, perfect lungs, kidneys, skin, and endocrine glands greatly improved the physical and chemical properties of the blood. While lower plants and animals are able to withstand wide fluctuations in physical and chemical properties, the latter attained extremely narrow limits in man alone, where body temperature is normal only within very few degrees. Beyond normal limits we will begin to shiver with cold or experience fever.

The tremendous narrowing of range of properties of the blood enabled the development of abstract thought, intelligence, coupled with fine movements of fingers to transmit thought, blooming in the manifestation of speech.

Since living organisms detached themselves from the earth to attain erect posture with mouthparts placed increasingly farther from the ground, we may safely attribute evolution of species to the gradual more organic nature of the food ingested, culminating in the use of fire to soften fibers, rendering food more palatable and digestible. For this reason we must use extreme care with the way foods are cooked when living organisms are prepared for food. The improper use of fire will reverse the evolutionary process in man and cause extinction.

CHAPTER XLIX

THE ORIGIN OF VARIATION OF SPECIES

One of the greatest problems facing medical science today is the origin of variation of species. If this could be solved we would eradicate birth defects forever from the face of the earth.

The solution of the cause of evolution enables me to state that the reason why species vary is because of slight variations in normal values of the blood, from conception until maturity.

Because all properties of the blood are governed by two important factors, oxygen and temperature , as shown by the classic experiment of the goldfish immersed in a beakerful of water whose temperature is lowered or raised, any study on species variation must take these two factors into consideration.

From *the moment of conception the embryo's life is closely tied to the mother's vital manifestations. Particularly during the first 2 months of pregnancy, abnormalities can occur. Blood flow to the embryo decreases when the mother's activities are excessive. It will also increase if the mother has fever, takes drugs or alcohol. While decreasing the flow causes defective growths, increasing the flow will cause monstrous growths.

* I wish to mention the great British physiologist Joseph Barcroft who said "there is an optimal concentration of oxygen in the blood plasma, and if there is any gross departure from this on either side, the higher functions of the brain will suffer."

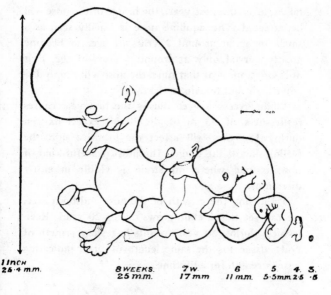

Fig 9 Series of 5 drawings illustrating the stages of growth from the end of the 3rd week to the end of the 8th.(From Keith, Human Embryology and Morphology)

After the 8th week of conception, structural abnormalities may not occur but growth in size can be affected. Increasing the flow can cause spontaneous abortion or permanent damage to nerve tissue.

The different nasal shapes seen all over the world show variations in oxygen intake after birth. While only the nostrils and base of nose are affected during the first year of life, when too much oxygen is intaken, after the first year, the bridge of the nose will be affected. The aquiline nose is usually seen as a small bump at around 2 years of age, to become greatly curved only at around 5 years of age. If it does not appear at that time, the nose will simply become high but remain straight.

While excess oxygen during the first year causes restlessness of 75 % of the brain, excess oxygen during 18 years will affect the intuitive side, the feeling side of the brain. The most peaceful kind of nose is one where no strain is visible in either directions.

Paralleling the growth of the nose and body size, we can see that a child grows during 20 years. Restlessness during 20 years results in restless growth of body tissue for the same length of time, indicating lesser strength for a lifetime.

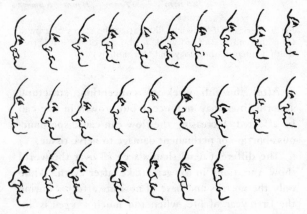

Fig. 10. Abnormal nasal profiles(From Berger)

Because of the great difference in nasal shapes between peoples, we can safely say it results from differences in cooking habits throughout the globe Thus if all peoples cooked in the same fashion, nasal shapes will tend to be more uniform. This is true within countries where similar food habits are the trend. Usually differences in nasal shapes can be found as one moves from one country to another where food habits are completely different.

While color of skin and curliness of hair result from higher environmental temperatures during the course of centuries, it is not wrong to say that if you want to remain fair and straight-haired, remain in the temperate zone, while if you want to become black and remain dark colored, live in environmental temperatures of 80° Fahrenheit and above. It is practically impossible to maintain the existence of dominant genes in temperate climates.

From the above, it is now possible to direct a child's growth through better food habits, thereby enhancing the growth of the brain and bodily tissues.

It is the trend today to build more and more tomblike structures, preventing the intake of air during the waking hours at work. This custom will force the breathing in of larger quantities of air during sleep, at night. In time, the nose will become affected, pushing the soft parts out of shape.

It is not wrong to say that when in adulthood the nose assumes a bulbous shape, we are on our way out with one foot in the grave. It is now time to think about building structures to allow all the fresh air within, for the number of people working in the area.

CHAPTER L

THE ABSOLUTE PRINCIPLE OF SCIENTIFIC DETERMINISM OF VITAL MANIFESTATIONS OF LIVING ORGANISMS

In his " INTRODUCTION TO THE STUDY OF EXPERIMENTAL MEDICINE" Claude Bernard repeatedly mentioned that determinism must exist in biological science, as in inorganic science.

Bodies of both kingdoms are dominated by a necessary determinism which ties them to certain purely physico-chemical conditions.

To Bernard the same principles govern both sciences. Manifestations of properties are tied to environmental conditions of temperature and humidity. In the organic kingdom it is among the lower animals that influences of temperature, humidity, light, heat are readily visible.

In the 1800's medical science was not advanced enough for a scientist to enounce an idea which could prove the existence of determinism. However Bernard felt that as medical science progresses we should arrive at this law underlying living organisms. To Bernard, to deny determinism signifies denying the biological sciences altogether. "An idea is a function of the time and place in which we live," said Bernard. When determinism will be found, it becomes a law, a scientific axiom, an absolute truth constituting an unchangeable criterion. To a practicing physician, this law should constantly be referred to during a lifelong career of diagnosis of illnesses.

The idea that enabled me to prove the law of determinism came to me in the summer of 1956, It can be stated as follows: Animals that feed upon food placed high in the scale of evolution are fast-moving animals. Animals that feed upon food low in the scale of evolution are slow-moving animals.

The above hypothesis was necessary for it is only by hypothesis, said Bernard, that one admits the absolute principle. While a hypothesis is a workable theory, it must be modified after submission to nature. One must always doubt oneself and one's interpretations until one arrives at a law with the greatest number of facts to support its proof.

Research begin in 1964 used Bernard's suggestions as a guideline. He said that in the manifestation of motion we must consider two bodies:

1. One which reacts or manifests the phenomenon.
2. Another which acts and plays the role of milieu to the first.

During the course of my research I often felt depressed and was tempted to renounce all further attempt to prove my hypothesis for there exists so many very small organisms in this world, rapid moving yet vegetarians. I clearly remember how I rapidly fingered through a book by Audubon, noting food habits and vital functions. It then dawned upon me that determinism can only be found among the larger organisms that eat only one type of food.

I was now ready to tackle the first of Bernard's suggestions: the body which reacts or manifests the phenomenon. In the following list gathered several years ago and never published, you will note that only a few organisms of each group are mentioned.

REGRESSION OF VITAL MANIFESTATIONS
ACCORDING TO FOOD HABITS

NAME	SPEED	SIZE	WEIGHT	FOOD HABITS
MAMMALS WHOSE PREY ARE MAMMALS				
Lion	50m/hr	9'	400-450 lbs	zebra & antelope
Tiger	50m/hr	9-9½'	400-450 lbs	small game to buff
Cheetah	70m/hr	7½'	100 lbs	musk oxen, deer, h
MAMMALS WHOSE PREY ARE FISH				
Common Dolphin	30 knots/ hr	8'		fish
MAMMALS WHOSE PREY ARE AQUATIC INVERTEBRATE				
Sperm whale	3-4 knots per hr	60'		Squid & cuttlefish
Stellar's Sea Lion	clumsy	13'		cuttlefish crustacea, small fish
MAMMALS WHOSE PREY ARE INSECTS				
Aadvark	clumsy gallop	6'		termites
Great Anteater	inoffensive	4'		termites & ants
Two-toed Anteater	movements sluggish	15'		Lermites

FRUIT - EATING MAMMALS

Gibbon	slow	3'	15 lbs	mainly fruit
Orang-utan	slow	4½'	200 lbs	mainly fruit
Three-toed sloth	1 mile in 6½hrs very slow	20'		leaves & fruit of Cecropia

LEAVES AND BUDS-EATING MAMMALS

Canadian porcupine	slow movement	3½'		buds & leaves, bark
Koala bear	tame & charming	2'		leaves of gum tree
Panda	slow & awkward on ground	2'		leaves & fruits

HERBIVOROUS MAMMALS

Malayan Tapir	defenceless	8'		vegetation, grass, leaves
White rhinoceros	inoffensive	12'	4 tons	grass
Yak	slow	6' 1"	200 lbs	sparse vegetation

MAMMALS THAT FEED UPON ALGAE

Manatee	slow	15'		underwater vegetation;
Dugong	slow	10'		underwater vegetation;

The above data show a gradual but definite decrease in speed of motion in larger animals as they feed upon lower organisms.

While it was simple to prove Bernard's first suggestion, it is much more difficult to prove his second point, as it is almost impossible to obtain values of blood properties for the above mentioned organisms. However we may assume that a definitely wider range of values of physical and chemical properties of the blood should be the trend among slow-moving animals.

The existence of determinism in the organic kingdom, shows how man's body can be affected by foods, especially when ill.

In my section on selection of foods for health I have used the principle of determinism for man's benefit. In general if you carefully choose your foods you will avoid drastic illnesses and even be able to help yourself in a most terminal state.

The principle of determinism should open up new fields in biology, such as a reclassification of Carl Linnaeus' system of classification in biology, where even today there exists much random placement of organisms.

CHAPTER LI

SOME TIPS TO A LONG LIFE

The other day I withnessed a strange incident.

A young man was repeatedly throwing a young woman over his shoulders. When she stood on her feet he made believe he was going to choke her. I was shocked beyond words. Calling him over I told him he shouldn't do that to her. I then asked whether she was his wife. He acquiesced. I further inquired whether he had done the same bouts to his first wife. He acknowledged. His first wife died after a year of marriage, beriddled with cancer at 18.

This young man had been at the marines and underwent such treatment from his fellow mates in the marine corps. When he married, he thought he'd play the same game with his wife. The poor girl was literally frightened to death, quickly developed cancer, became pregnant. The baby was removed from her womb before term, for fear the mother might die. Shortly after, she died. The young man quickly remarried and continued with the same game on his second young wife.

The above case is an extreme example of a total lack of understanding, love and terderness, from a young husband, mostly due to his own ignorance. In general, when we must constantly live with a mate, extreme understanding and kindness should exist between two people. The fact that one must see each other at all times, elbowing one other constantly, only respect toward one other's feelings, awareness of one's needs can ensure a long life to both parties.

Ever so often an individual has the right to be alone and should be allowed to do so. Sometimes one has the desire to eat a particular food. One should not criticize such habits.

Many people believe it the greatest thing in the world to have a lot of friends, yet personal experience and assertion from others prove that envy, desire, injurious statements exist between so-called friends. In general it is better to have one or two very good friends than a whole gamut of worthless friends, eager to take advantage of your good fortune or hurt your feelings when you are down and out.

In many families today, both adults and children alike believe that fear is an interesting passion to arouse. For this reason parents and brothers and sisters are the targets. They are frightened for kicks. Fear as we all know, is one of the most dangerous passions to arouse. Continued fright can cause cancer or dysfunction of any of the regulatory organs. We must learn never to frighten anyone for the fun of it!

Another factor concerns sleeping habits. Most people today will wake someone up without any regard. One must never, but never awaken anyone who is asleep. The fact alone that one sleeps simply shows that the regulatory organs are in need of a great supply of blood at that moment. It is best to leave one alone and never to awaken anyone who is in a deep sleep. In an emergency if one must awaken someone by all means, it should be done only by gentle stroking of the skin or hair, until one's eyes open up. You can develop intense hatred toward the one who dares awaken you in a sudden fashion.

In general a long life can be achieved by doing things at a slow pace. We can learn to observe some of the giant turtles who live several hundred years. Slow movements are more inducive to a long life than quick, jerky actions. You can visualize the slow movement of blood to opened capillaries when life's actions are slow.

We must also learn to use life's forces with care. Expenditure of extreme energy over a long period of time can definitely lead to a shortened life.

Sensitivity to dangerous situations is the most impotant safeguard in life. Let your feelings tell you what you should do or avoid and follow your instinct. No one in this world knows you better than yourself.

CONCLUSION

Now that you have come to the end of this guide you will probably exclaim "Why, if everything I do kills red blood cells then I'd be better off doing nothing all day long!" Which in a way is exactly what lower organisms do. Because we have a brain that can think, we must do something otherwise we'd be bored to death. This guide is supposed to help you to preserve your energies as you work. It should help you control your body at all times despite the most adverse conditions, to preserve it in any event of disaster.

Hua To, famous surgeon of AD220 in China, said that the body must work but not to its utmost capacity. Motion helps the digestion of food. increases the circulation of blood through arteries and veins in all directions, so that no diseases appear.

He stresses the importance of stretching, pulling limbs and joints, imitating the tiger, the stag, the bear, the monkey and the bird. He believes that if we imitate these animals in our movements, we can remain nimble and young for life.

SOME DELICIOUS RECIPES FOR EVERYONE

Steamed fish

 1 small whole fish or the head end or tail end of a striped bass, soy sauce, garlic powder, ginger, wine, jam or sugar, salt.

 Brush a little oil in frying pan. Heat till fuming hot. Drop fish in pan and brown it until skin is dark and paper thin on both sides. Place it in a shallow dish. Add seasonings. Place it in a hot steamer where fire is medium high. Steam fish until aroma is perceptible or when a fork pokes through (around 15 min.) Place some bits of scallions on fish before removing from steamer. Serve.

 This recipe may be steamed plain and served with a sweet and sour sauce.

Pot roast. (This may be used for short ribs or beef, lamb neck bones) 1 lb of pork neck bones or spare ribs in inch size pieces, soy sauce, garlic, ginger, wine, jam or sugar, salt, 1 onion cut up.

Brown pieces of meat with bone in a frying pan. Drop in a large pot. Add onion, seasonings. Cover. Turn heat on low(as low as possible) and simmer until meat is mealy and tender(about 2 hours), at which point the aroma is perceptible. Serve.

Shrimp and scallions.

1 lb of giant shrimps, 3 scallions, seasonings, corn starch. Peel and devein shrimps. Cut them in small pieces. Add seasonings, a tablespoonful or corn starch. Mix well.

In a pan, brush a little oil or fat. Heat. Over low flame stir shrimps until they are done and aroma is perceptible. Add bits of scallions and stir a few more minutes. Serve.

This recipe may be varied with chicken breast meat cut up, pork chops cut up into bits, beefsteak cut up paper thin. The vegetables may be varied with green pepper, squash, mushrooms. etc.

Shia Chiao or shrimp dumplings.

1/2 lb of wheat starch. Pour very hot but not boiling water on starch, stirring constantly until a hard dough is formed. Knead dough and shape it into a long sausage. Place it in a hot steamer and steam for exactly five minutes. Remove from steamer. Add one teaspoon of butter or lard to dough. Knead well.

Place inch size pieces of dough on board, flouring board with wheat starch as needed. Roll out and place the following filling in it.

Filling: 1 lb of shrimp cut into pieces. A few bamboo shoots or water chestnuts, or simply use American cabbage in tiny squares and scallions. Add two teaspoons of lard to mixture, salt and garlic to taste. Place a teaspoonful of filling in rolled out dough, wrap it up in the shape of a bonnet. When 4 are ready, place them on a small dish and steam for 15 minutes. Serve.

Roast Duck: Marinate a thawed duck overnight in ginger, garlic, soy sauce, wine, jam and other spices, The next day, place duck without seasonings in a baking dish at 400° in oven. When it sizzles, take it out, remove fat. Turn duck around.

Keep doing so every time it sizzles, for about 2 hours, reducing heat gradually until all duck's fat is rent and duck appears dark brown. At this point place seasonings, neck, gizzard, liver and heart in baking dish and cook duck in low heat until a fork pokes through easily and you perceive the aroma of cooked meat. Serve. (Cooking time: around 3 hrs.)

Pork Dumplings:

Filling:

1 lb ground pork	¼ cup water
2 green peppers	1 tbsp soy sauce
2 eggs	1 tbsp wine
4 scallions	grated ginger,
1 bunch parsley	1 tsp salt
1 tbsp cornstarch	garlic and other
2 zucchinis	seasonings

Chop all ingredients very fine. Mix altogether.

Skin: To ½ lb flour, add ½ cup corn starch and enough water to make a hard dough. Add salt and knead. When hard, add a lump of butter and knead again. Refrigerate.

Make dumplings by using a broosmsize rolling pin.

Take a large piece of dough. Roll it out on corn-starch floured surface. Cut round pieces of dough with a large cup. Roll with pin again. When very thin, fill each piece with the above filling. When half a dozen dumplings are ready, drop them in a pot of boiling water and cook until water boils. Add a little cold water and boil it once more. Serve.

The dough may also be made with boiling water.

BIBLIOGRAPHICAL REFERENCES

1. Barcroft, Joseph, FEATURES IN THE ARCHITECTURE OF PHYSIOLOGICAL FUNCTION, Cambridge University Press, N.Y., 1934.
2. Barcroft, Joseph, THE BRAIN AND ITS ENVIRONMENT, Yale University Press, New Haven, 1938.
3. Bauer, Julius, M.D., FA.C.P. THE PERSON BEHIND THE DISEASE, Grune & Stratton, N.Y. & London, 1956.
4. Bernard, Claude, LE CAHIER ROUGE, Translated by Roger Guillemin and Lucienne Guillemin, and Hebbel Hoff, Schenkman Publishing Company, 1967.
5. Bernard, Claude, INTRODUCTION A L'ETUDE DE LA MEDECINE EXPERIMENTALE, Flammarion, Editeur, Paris, France, 1952.
6. Best, C.H. and Taylor, W.B., THE LIVING BODY, Chapman and Hall Ltd, 4th Edition, London, 1959.
7. Cannon, Walter. B.,THE WISDOM OF THE BODY, W.W. Norton and Co. Second Edition, New York, 1963.
8. Diehl, H.S. and Dahlrymple, W., HEALTHFUL LIVING, 9th Edition, McGraw Hill Book Co., New York, 1973.
9. Ho, Betty Yü-Lin, HOW TO STAY HEALTHY A LIFETIME WITHOUT MEDICINES, Juvenescent Research Corporation, New York, 1979.
10. Kinsey, A.C., Pomeroy, W.B., Martin, C.E. Belhard, P.H., SEXUAL BEHAVIOR IN THE HUMAN FEMALE W.B. Saunders Co., Phila., 1953.

11. Keith, A., HUMAN EMBRYOLOGY AND MOR-
PHOLOGY, W. Wood & Co., 5th Edition, Baltimo-
re, 1933.
12. Kraus, B.S.,THE BASIS OF HUMAN EVOLUTION,
Harper and Bros., New York, 1964.
13. Krogh, August, THE ANATOMY AND PHYSIO-
LOGY OF CAPILLARIES, Revised Edition, Yale
University Press, New Haven. 1929.
14. Portmann, Adolf, NEW PATHS IN BIOLOGY,
Edited by Ruth Nanda Anshen, World Perspectives,
Volume 20, Harper and Row, 1964.
15. Prosser, C.L. and Brown, F.A., COMPARATIVE
ANIMAL PHYSIOLOGY, 2nd Edition, W.B. Saunders, Phila., 1950.
16. Routh, J.I., FUNDAMENTALS OF INORGANIC
ORGANIC AND BIOLOGICAL CHEMISTRY, W.B.
Saunders, Phila., 1954.
17. THE ENCYCLOPEDIA BRITANNICA, W. Benton,
Chicago, 1969.
18. Veith, Ilza, Translated by, THE YELLOW EMPER—
OR'S CLASSIC OF INTERNAL MEDICINE, University of California Press, Berkeley, California,
1072.
19. Walter, H.E., THE HUMAN SKELETON, Macmil-
lan, New York, 1918.